HIIT

The Fastest Way to Get Ripped and Maximize
Your Workout

(Fastest Way to Burn Fat and Lose Weight!)

Douglas Hooper

Published by Andrew Zen

Douglas Hooper

All Rights Reserved

HIIT: The Fastest Way to Get Ripped and Maximize Your Workout (Fastest Way to Burn Fat and Lose Weight!)

ISBN 978-1-989965-98-6

Legal & Disclaimer

The information contained in this book is not designed to replace or take the place of any form of medicine or professional medical advice. The information in this book has been provided for educational and entertainment purposes only.

The information contained in this book has been compiled from sources deemed reliable, and it is accurate to the best of the Author's knowledge; however, the Author cannot guarantee its accuracy and validity and cannot be held liable for any errors or omissions. Changes are periodically made to this book. You must consult your doctor or get professional medical advice before using any of the suggested remedies, techniques, or information in this book.

Upon using the information contained in this book, you agree to hold harmless the Author from and against any damages, costs, and expenses, including any legal fees potentially resulting from the application of any of the information provided by this guide. This disclaimer applies to any damages or injury caused by the use and application, whether directly or indirectly, of any advice or information presented, whether for breach of contract, tort, negligence, personal injury, criminal intent, or under any other cause of action.

You agree to accept all risks of using the information presented inside this book. You need to consult a professional medical practitioner in order to ensure you are both able and healthy enough to participate in this program.

Table of Contents

Introduction

This book provides proven strategies and steps to tone up and slim down without going to the gym.

I am excited to share with you High Intensity Interval training (or H.I.I.T. I'm excited to introduce you to High Intensity Interval Training (or H.I.I.T. for short). It is simple and will help you lose weight for many years. You will learn the proven methods bodybuilders, crossfitters and others use to stay lean all year. This book will teach you how to do HIIT, as well as the principles behind it. It covers everything, from the basics of HIIT programming to how to program a simple HIIT workout at your home. You should be able to create your own HIIT program by the end of the book! The book's purpose is to teach you how to use HIIT without a gym. Most of the exercises will focus on basic bodyweight movements.

Chapter 1: Benefits Of Hiit

HIIT is not for the weak, but the benefits from this exercise program make the pain worth it. These are the benefits of HIIT:

Quick and Doable

One of the best things about HIIT is that it is accessible everywhere at any time. One does not need any gym equipment to do the program, plus it only requires a few minutes per day. Even if you are in the office, a hotel room or you are on vacation, you can easily spare 30 minutes of your time to undergo HIIT.

It increases metabolism

Since it constantly pushes the body to the limit, the body adjusts to endure longer and harder training exercises. Another benefit of HIIT is a person continues to burn fat after training because of EPOC.

Improved insulin capacity

HIIT teaches the body to burn glucose instantly instead of reaching into stored fats. Whatever is eaten before a workout is automatically burned before the body uses stored fats.

It has an anabolic effect

The intense workout encourages muscle formation and fat loss. It may seem the workout time is shorter than in normal aerobic training, but the body is able to burn more calories over an hour of training and lifting.

In a study made, two groups trained at the same time. The traditional aerobic group exercised for 15 weeks and burned 35-40% of targeted calories while the group that practiced interval training exercised for 10 weeks and burned 5 times as many calories as the aerobic group.

No equipment required

HIIT is cheap to do. It doesn't require any gym equipment, though you may use one if you want. HIIT training can be done outdoors, or indoors doing stationary intense exercises.

It curbs hunger

When the body makes use of glucose more efficiently, hunger pangs are less likely to happen. After an intense workout, the body reaches first to available glucose then to stored fats. Even though you've worked out profusely, you won't feel physical hunger.

It slows down aging

HIIT triggers the production of Human Growth Hormone (HGH). HGH is responsible for continuous calorie burning after training. It also slows the aging process, which makes people look and feel younger.

It's easy to track

HIIT processes and results are easy to keep track of. It only takes a digital timer to monitor your workout and rest period. The results are easily visible, especially muscle formation. Within 6-8 weeks of HIIT, trainers appeared to have toned bodies and less body fat.

No loose skin

HIIT does not cause loose skin or arm flab when fat is burned. Only muscle formation occurs unlike in other exercise programs that burn fat but leave the skin loose.

It has rest periods

Unlike other training programs, HIIT allows the person to 'rest' or slow during the course of training. Resting is an important part of HIIT; it allows the person to recover for a short while. These short rests are essential for the person to continue with the remaining exercises.

It's a time-saver

People are busy juggling their personal lives and career demands; most of the time exercise or gym time is taken for granted. HIIT is ideal and convenient for busy people. It is doable anywhere, and takes only a few minutes. People won't have any excuse not to be able to undergo training anymore.

High efficiency

Whether you're a full-time mom, a working student or a busy man, HIIT can still work for your busy schedule. Surely, you'll be able to do this because it doesn't require a lot of time. It works effectively, too, if you have to attend to an event where you need to have a desired shape. Your aerobic capability will also be enhanced in 2 weeks of high intensity intervals.

Less body fats

The amount of calories this workout will burn depends on your size, gender and health condition. The usual HIIT session for beginners can burn 7-12 calories a minute. You probably burn 152-252 calories on the entire routine. If you're a heavyweight person, expect to burn more than the estimated number of calories

Chapter 2: Hiit Procedures

Like many other exercise routines, HIIT is done in sessions to easily schedule when it's done or track progress. While the approaches differ from individual to individual, they follow a basic pattern. The session starts with warm-up exercise, then followed by the alternating reiterations of high and medium to low intensity exercise, and then finally ends with a cool-down exercise. The periods of high intensity are done at maximum or near maximum exertion. The medium to low intensity periods are done with about 50% or lower. The alternating repetitions vary greatly, but typically it consists of at least 3 repetitions with as short as 10 seconds for each of the high intensity exercise.

The individual's cardiovascular development level influences the type of exercises done by the individual. The recovery exercise may be any slow movement like simply walking. The usual high intensity workout is a sprint. There is no strict formula but one commonly used is a ratio of 1:2 – intense work: recovery. For example, if the session involves between a 15- and 20-second sprint, the alternating recovery will be a 30-40 second walk or slow jog.

An HIIT session can last from 4 to 30 minutes, making it shorter than most types of workout.

Known Regimens

Throughout the establishment and development of HIIT, different regimens came out.

Peter Coe Regimen

The Peter Coe regimen was employed in the 1970s by its namesake Peter Coe, an athletic coach, when he set sessions for Sebastian Coe, his son. His regimen was inspired by principles promoted by Woldemar Gerschler, a university professor and German coach, and Per-Olof Astrand, a Swedish physiologist. The Peter Coe regimen involved fast 200 meter runs – each speedy run separated by recovery periods lasting 30 seconds.

Tabata Regimen

In 1996, Professor Izumi Tabata and his colleagues conducted a study that initially involved Olympic speed skaters. In the study, they performed a 20-second period of high intensity exercise followed by a rest of 10 seconds. This cycle is continuously repeated for 4 minutes for a total of 8 cycles. Subjects perform 4 sessions of this a week. Tabata gave this the label IE1 protocol.

The HIIT version based from this study is called the Tabata regimen. The regimen was formulated because of the positive results from the study. The subjects performing the HIIT had their results compared with a group of other athletes who performed steady-state training five times a week. Their gains were similar, with the overall gain higher for the HIIT group. However the HIIT group obviously had to spend a much shorter time on their training regime, making it beneficial. Moreover, anaerobic capacity improvements were only found on the HIIT group.

Gibala Regimen

In Canada, Professor Martin Gibala, together with his team in McMaster

University, has conducted research on highly intense exercise already going on for a good number of years. In 2009, their study involved students who did sessions each with 3-minute warm up, 60-second high intensity exercise and then 75-second recovery. The work-rest cycle was repeated about 8-12 times. The routine is sometimes called "The Little Method". The subjects performed this HIIT variation three times a week. The subjects' gains were similar to subjects who performed steady-state exercises five times per week. This form of HIIT is still physically demanding, but the protocol can be done by the average person using only an exercise bike.

In 2011, Gibala and his team released a variation with less intensity of the regimen they used. The objective is to provide a similar but gentler HIIT version for those who hadn't exercised for more than a year. The variation goes like: 3 minutes warm up, 10 cycles of 60-second work using peak power at 60%, with 60-second recovery, and closes with a cool down of 5-minute duration.

Timmons Regimen

Systems biology professor Jamie Timmons at University of Loughborough is an advocate of using few short spurts of exercise with flat-out levels of intensity. February of 2012, his regimen was shown to be used by Michael J. Mosley through a BBC Horizon program. This particular regimen consisted of three cycles with 20 seconds of maximum effort cycling bursts with 2 minutes of gentle pedaling. The session was thrice a week, adding up to a total of 3 minutes intense workout each week, adding the warm-up and the recovery time. In the said run by Mosley, quantifiable benefits to health were recorded; substantial improvement in insulin sensitivity included.

Next...

The regimens described above are just some common forms of HIIT. The variations are endless but you will find most of them originated from these four regimens.

In the next chapters, you will find some characteristics of HIIT that make it an ideal workout for many people.

Chapter 3: Starting Hiit

Are you old enough to have experienced reading the Choose Your Own Adventure series of books back in the 1980s and 1990s? If you are and if you actually loved those books, chances are high that you'll also love HIIT if only for the pleasure of being able to "cook up" your own workout programs. As mentioned earlier, the HIIT program is based on just one major tenet: alternate short bursts of high-intensity exercise with longer periods of rest or low-intensity exercises. Further, I also mentioned that the terms "high-intensity" and "low-intensity" are relative and can be adjusted accordingly. Together, these 2 characteristics make the HIIT program one where you can exercise a great deal of creative control – just like the Choose Your Own Adventure series.

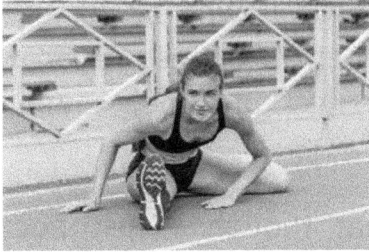

Beginning HIITs

If you're new to this, it may be quite challenging to determine how short and long your high-intensity and low-intensity intervals must be, considering that there's really no "benchmark" or "gold standard' for it. Fortunately, a good guide for your durations is the Tabata protocol or method, which I mentioned earlier. There's a reason why it's one of the most – if not the most – popular HIIT method or protocol – it seems to work for most people who do HIIT. As such, it's a good place to start – 10 seconds of high intensity effort followed by 20 seconds of low intensity effort or rest, repeated for a minimum period of time, say 5 or 10 minutes.

Just a caveat though – just because it works for most people doesn't mean you should stick to it if you find it doesn't work for you. Listen to your body – extend and reduce the high and low-intensity durations, respectively if it's too "light" or reduce and extend the high and low intensity durations, respectively, if it's too intense for you at the start.

And just a gentler reminder: do not neglect the habit of doing dynamic stretches for at least 5 minutes prior to your HIIT sessions and static stretches for cooling down afterward in order to minimize your risks for injuries as well as to maximize your muscles' recovery.

Time after Time

Anything worth doing or achieving requires sufficient time. There are no shortcuts – trust the process as the former general manager of the Philadelphia 76ers in the NBA would say. If you attempt to shortcut the process, you may pay dearly for it with burnout or worse, injuries.

When working out using HIIT, you will have to start where you are – with what you perceive as "maximum effort." Performing 20 pushups in 30 seconds may bring you closer to the edge of passing out but for a Navy SEAL, that's probably low-intensity. Don't compare your "maximum effort" to others' because the moment you do, you'd have lost all objectivity and put yourself at great risk of doing too much too soon.

One of the best ways to start building up your high-intensity tolerance is by doing 5 minutes of HIIT at the beginning. If it's too easy, then extend it to 10 minutes and so on. Better to err on the side of caution, as the smartest people in the planet would often say.

Don't be intimidated

While it's true that the HIIT is not a program for sissies and wimps, it doesn't mean you have to be ultra-fit and strong to start. The reason you – and everybody else for that matter – would like to get in on the program is to become much stronger, fitter and energetic! So, that being said, you need not fear the result of a hundred HIIT sessions. Okay, just a few sessions for starters. As mentioned earlier, start where you are, not where others are or where others expect you to start. From there, start to gradually build up your ability to do more and more high-intensity work. Better yet, start by enlisting the services of a personal trainer until you already have a very good grasp of the program, in which case you can go on your own and make your own HIIT way.

So again, do not be scared of HIIT or be overly concerned with other people's fitness or expectations of you. Start where you are, be consistent and you'll gradually get there. What's important is you get there, not how fast you do.

It Gets Easier

Because of the program's ability to burn so many calories – and consequently body fat – while exercising for a relatively shorter period of time, HIIT is one of the most popular physical training programs around. By using exercise or intensity intervals, you push your body to gradually increase your metabolism via purposeful decrease and increase in heart rate, a.k.a., alternating low and high-intensity exercises. And as part of increasing your body's metabolic rate, you'll be able to train for managing your personal energy systems better too. For example, if you simply ran for 1 hour straight, you may be able to cover about 7 kilometers as an average runner before hitting the so-called "wall." But if you use what's known in running circles as the Galloway or "Run-Walk" method, you'll be able to extend your running time to more than 1 hour, maintain your top running speed for longer too, and cover more distance in the process. Why? Because by taking frequent walking breaks regardless of how energetic you feel at the end of a particular interval, you manage your energy much better and extend it further.

But as with all good things, the HIIT program's not perfect. In particular, it may be more detrimental than beneficial for you if you have a pre-existing serious cardio vascular condition. In this case, it's better to check with a doctor first before you even consider doing HIIT. Also, if you're currently nursing an injury or have some other physical or medical condition that may be worsened by the grueling exercise sessions in HIIT, either you'll have to check with your doctor first or skip HIIT altogether. Better safe than dead.

Your Daily break

Another thing you'll need to keep in mind if you'd like to maximize your chances of achieving your dream body, getting uber fit, and looking years younger than your age is to respect your body by giving it enough rest in between your HIIT sessions. In particular, do not perform HIIT daily. Why?

First of all, it's not your usual exercise routine – it's high intensity, remember? As such, your body will need a longer period of time to recover from the onslaught and a 24-hour rest period isn't enough. And speaking of 24 hours...

The second reason why you shouldn't have your daily HIITs is that on average, muscles need about 48 hours of rest prior to being worked out again. So if you plan to optimize the physical benefits of HIIT, the most you can do them is 4 times a week. More than that, you increase your risk of injuries and burnout.

Optimizing Your HIITs

To summarize this chapter, keep the following things in mind as you start HIITing your way to a fit, strong and energetic body in order to maximize your results:

● Take It Slow: If you start by using the Tabata protocol and find it's still a bit above what your body can handle, don't hesitate to extend your resting or low-intensity interval. Only once you're able to properly handle the high-intensity nature of your initial HIITs should you increase the duration of your high intensity intervals and reduce that of the low-intensity or resting ones.

● Always Warm Up: I can't overemphasize the value of warming up properly with dynamic stretches. Your body needs to be primed for the fast and intense HIIT exercises to which you'll subject it because otherwise, you risk injuring your major joints, i.e., the wrists, neck, hips, shoulders, ankles, elbows and legs. In particular, do a lot of circular movements before shifting to jumping jacks or a light jog to complete your dynamic stretching or warm up.

● Monitor Your Repetitions: To monitor your progress, you'll need to rely on something more than just "feel." You will need something objective to evaluate your progress or lack of it. Repetitions – coupled with time – are as objective as objective monitoring can be for your HIIT progress. So if you're doing 20 reps for 20 seconds on the first couple of days, you must be able to either do more reps for the same time or increase your high-intensity durations for the same exercises after a month to say you've progressed.

● Use A HIIT-Friendly Timer: Also called an interval timer, it's going to take a whole lot of mental burden and distraction off your shoulders when you perform HIIT workouts. As if doing HIIT isn't already difficult enough for a beginner, what more if you add the mental burden of having to always look at the clock while performing your exercises to make sure you stick to your interval protocols. In this day and age of smartphones and apps, you can use an app like Deltaworks Interval Timer to help you keep to your chosen protocol or interval durations. With apps like this, all you'll need to do is set your protocol's parameters (interval times), activate and go!

● Avoid Doing HIIT Daily: As mentioned earlier, you'll need to give your body enough time for rest and recuperation, especially if you're a newbie to the program. And if you remember, the guideline is 48 hours. In between, you can do other types of training like biking, swimming, or Pilates and Yoga.

● KISS or Keep It Short and Sweet: An interval, for HIIT purposes, shouldn't go beyond 1 minute to be optimal. It's because you can only push your body to the max for 60 seconds or less. If you can push it above 60 seconds, it means you haven't really exerted maximum effort – you'll need to exert more effort to ensure that you're temporarily spent in 60 seconds or less. If you're having a hard time figuring it out, refer back to chapter the section on intensity levels in the previous chapter, i.e., the talk test.

● Always Better Together: When working out with a partner, you have someone to push you to your limits (or even beyond) and if you don't give it your all, someone to kick your butt! Either way, having someone train with you increases your chances of giving it all you got all the way and consequently, maximize your HIIT results.

Chapter 4: Hiit Treadmill Workouts

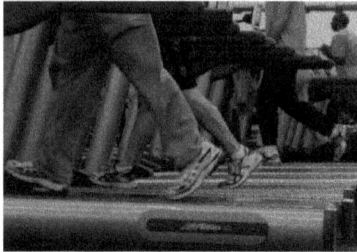

HIIT Treadmill Workout Version 1

Step 1: - Warm up

Begin with a warm up on your treadmill. Set the incline at a slow pace and walk or jog for 5 minutes to encourage the blood to flow to the muscles while getting your body ready for the higher intensity activities. While warming up, try to keep your elbows slightly above the heart position.

Step 2: - Sprint

Increase the treadmill speed so that you can sprint for about 30 seconds. You should be aiming for a 90-percent maximum heart rate until you reach a point where you are unable to talk.

Step 3: - Slow down

After 30 seconds, reduce your sprint speed to a fast-paced walk or a light jog and do this for 2 minutes. Your recovery/slow intensity time should be at least 3-5 times your total high-intensity duration. In case you had pushed your high intensity interval to the maximum, a slow walk will be necessary.

Step 4: - High Intensity

Switch to another high intensity sprint for another 30 seconds before switching back to a slow-paced walk. Alternate the high and low intensity workouts until you reach your 15-minute goal.

You can incorporate some 15 to 20 sets of squats to work on your quadriceps or hold dumbbells if you are in good shape already.

HIIT Treadmill Workout Version 2

This second High Intensity Interval Training workout involves a combination of sprint and strength. During this workout, you will pair lower body exercises (pistol squats, squats, plyometric box jumps or leg press) with treadmill sprints.

Step 1: - Warm up

Set the treadmill at easy-moderate pace and warm up for about 5 minutes to prepare the body for the high intensity workouts.

Step 2: - Sprint

Set the treadmill speed to a pace that you are comfortable with but also one that pushes you to the limit. Sprint for 60 seconds.

Step 3: - Lower body workouts

After the sprint, get off your treadmill and do 10 to 15 lower body workout reps of your choice. You can choose to combine two or three but make sure they are pushing your body to the limit.

Step 4: - Rest and resume the Sprint

Once you are done with the lower body exercises, rest for about 30 seconds and then get back to the treadmill. Increase the speed and sprint for 30 seconds before slowing down to recover.

The strength exercises and sprints can be repeated in alternating cycles for 4 to 6 times.

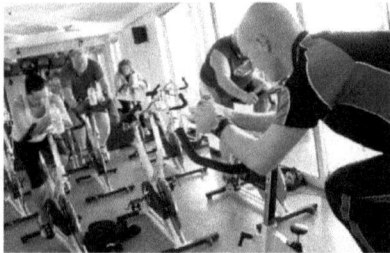

HIIT cycle workouts

The secret behind effective HIIT cycling workouts is in the increased RPM (Revolutions per Minute) or leg speed against suitable resistance levels (incline or gear) so as to increase your heart rate to the maximum thus leading to an amazing cardiovascular response. The best thing will be to increase the surge and perform the workouts for short intervals thus maximizing the benefits. However, always make sure you have sufficient resting intervals especially if you are a HIIT Cycling workout beginner.

HIIT Cycle Workout 1

Step 1: -Warm up

Begin by performing a 3-minute warm up on your stationary bike at approximately 65 percent heart rate.

Step 2: Explode into cycling

Explode into hard, fast cycling for about 30 seconds, and then slow down again for about 15 seconds. Repeat the hard and fast cycling interval and then enter into the recovery interval. Repeat for 7-8 rounds.

Step 3: - Cool down

Conclude by performing a 3-minute cool down cycling at a slow and comfortable pace.

HIIT Cycling workout 2

Step 1: - Warm up

Start by warming up at a maximum 65-percent heart rate for about 3 minutes.

Step 2: - Intensified cycling

Accelerate your cycling momentum as hard as possible and go for 1 kilometer. Reduce the intensity to a comfortable pace and do this until you reach a 125-RPM heart rate. Repeat the intervals for 15 minutes or more based on your endurance level.

Step 3: - Cool down

Cycle slowly in a pace you are comfortable with to allow your body to cool down.

HIIT Cycling Workout 3

Step 1: - Warm up

Start by performing a 3-minute warm up session at 65 percent heart rate.

Step 2: - Intensified pedaling

Push the pedal as hard as possible for an interval of 30 seconds before slowing down for a recovery period of 30 seconds. Repeat the pedaling but make sure your RPM is set at more than 120.

Step 3: - Cool down

Slow down the pedaling to a comfortable pace and go for a 3-minute interval to help you cool down.

Sprint intervals

Sprint intervals offer you a great interval workout to achieve your desired shape. Sprint intervals also offer cardio respiratory benefits and the best strength training within a short time. You can craft a calorie-blasting, fun routine by alternating between explosive high intensity sprint intervals and low intensity bodyweight workouts.

Sprint Interval Workout Steps

Start your workout with a 20-second jogging or paced walk interval before bursting into a fast sprint for 10 seconds. Slow down for a recovery period of 30 seconds which you should spend jogging or walking slowly. After 30 seconds, switch to another interval of fast, hard sprint for 10 seconds and then rest. Repeat the intervals until you reach your 15-minute target.

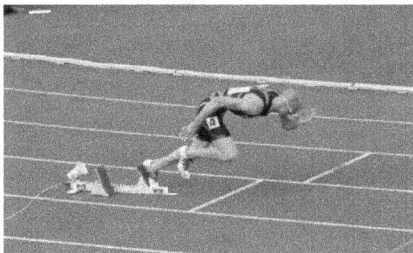

Advanced Sprint HIIT Workout

Step 1: Warm Up
Have a 4-minute warm-up by simply jogging at 50 percent effort.

Step 2: First workout interval

Go for an all-out sprint interval for 30 seconds.

Step 3: Recovery

Rest for 10 seconds by just walking or jogging lightly just to recover the oxygen deficit and refill your gas tank.

Repeat these intervals interchangeably for 15 minutes and finish by simply doing a cool down interval of light jogging (about 50 percent).

You can do this HIIT sprint workout for up to 8 weeks but always make sure you are monitoring your heart rate throughout the workout so as to be sure that you are reaching the desired intensity levels.

HIIT elliptical workouts

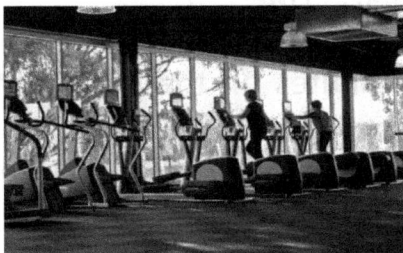

High Intensity Interval Training Elliptical workouts are the buzz of cardio training today. The workouts normally combine high intensity short sessions of exercises with complete rest or low intensity exercise sessions. If you find the 30-60-minute continuous cardio exercises to be boring and hard to keep up with, then you will fall in love with the 15-minute HIIT Elliptical workouts. The workouts provide amazing benefits compared to the long, traditional cardio workouts.

How to perform 15-minute HIIT Elliptical workouts?

Step 1: - Warm Up

Take 3-5 minutes on the elliptical trainer with an easy resistance and incline. This prepares your body for the workout intervals ahead.

Step 2: - Workout

Set your first workout interval at an incline of 5 and resistance of 5. Remain at this rate for up to 2 minutes. Remain at the incline of 5 but increase resistance to 10 and remain there for 1 minute.

Switch to the next interval, turn resistance to 5, and incline to 7 for 2 minutes. Increase the resistance to 10 while incline remains at 7 for 1 minute and then increase the resistance to 10 while incline remains at 7.

Increase the momentum, set resistance at 7 and incline at 9 and workout for 2 minutes before switching to a resistance of 12 and an incline of 9 for 1 minute.

With the incline at 9, change the resistance to level 7 and remain in that position for 2 minutes before switching gears to a resistance of 12 while incline remains at 9. Stay at resistance 12 and incline 9 for 1 minute.

Finish your 15-minute HIIT Elliptical workout by setting the resistance at 9 and incline at 11 for 2 minutes. Switch to a resistance of 14 and maintain an incline of 11 for 1 minute.

Cool down with an easy resistance and incline for 3-5 minutes.

Instructions:

During the one-minute intervals, you should give the workout everything you have got since these are your high-intensity intervals. Ease the momentum during the 2-minute intervals for recovery. You can repeat the previous resistance levels or modify the settings in such a way that you will be comfortable but still apply some pressure on your body.

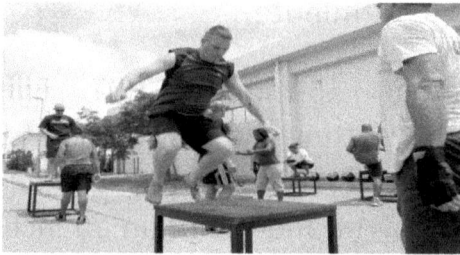

HIIT Cardio workouts

Short HIIT cardio workouts can help blast more calories and fat than the traditional cardio workouts that many people find boring and dreadful. There are different

High Intensity Interval Training cardio workouts you can try including the following: -

Kettlebell Swings

The HIIT Cardio workouts can help work your hamstrings, back muscles, oblique/abdominal muscles and glutes perfectly well. They also help in engaging the core muscles and strengthening knees and hips. During the concentric swing, muscle activation rises up before transitioning to complete relaxation during the eccentric phase. Always choose your weights carefully since you won't be going for a one rep max.

How to do kettlebell swings?

Step 1: - Warm-up

Jump rope moderately for 5 minutes or opt for a 10-minute jog or brisk walk.

Step 2: - Workout interval

Go for 5 sets of all out swings in 10 to 30 second intervals before switching to recovery/rest intervals of 45 to 60 seconds in-between the sets.

Step 3- Cool down

Cool down by taking a 10-minute jog/ brisk walk or jump rope moderately.

Alternative HIIT Cardio workouts

Power Knee Drives

Always start your workouts with a warm up interval to prepare the body for the high intensity exercises. This always helps the body to adapt and cooperate without breaking down.

Workout Steps

Start your interval from a front lunge position. Bend your knee to a 90-degree position while bending your opposite arm in from of the chest as though you are sprinting. Push the back knee up before exploding off with the standing leg and use your arm to propel your body off the floor. This should take about 15 seconds. Rest for 30 seconds and then return to your starting position but switch the legs. Continue in this position for 15 seconds, rest and then keep alternating until you reach your goal.

Circuit Workouts

You can also combine different workouts in short intervals of 30 seconds each according to the following two circuits given below.

Circuit 1

Start with a warm up session of 3-5 minutes. You can either jog or walk briskly.

Go for burpees for 30 seconds and then rest for 30 more seconds (Can walk or jog lightly) before switching to mountain climbers for 30 more seconds. Take a 30-second rest break before doing a squat-jump interval for 30 seconds. Rest for 30 seconds and then repeat these same workouts afresh until you reach your goal.

Circuit 2

Do turbo lunges for 30 seconds followed by line jumps for 30 seconds. Switch to boxer kicks for 30 seconds. Take 30 seconds to rest between each workout and then repeat 10 times.

Doing HIIT Workouts right

The secret behind successful HIIT is in how you do your workouts. Instead of going for steady-paced aerobic workouts, that takes up to 30 minutes or one hour, you will be alternating intense workout intervals with slower recovery intervals. However, the advantage is that you burn more calories during and after you are through with your sessions. The process of burning calories even after the workouts, normally known as EPOC (Excessive Post-exercise Oxygen Consumption) plays an important role in the weight loss equation and this is something that can only be achieved through HIIT as opposed to the traditional steady-paced exercises since it raises the heart rate to the maximum.

To avoid the risk of injuries and burnout, it is always good to start your workout sessions with a short warm up which should last for at least 5 minutes or so. To maximize your HIIT effectiveness, always consider these essential tips: -

Start gradually and increase the frequency slowly

The aim is to achieve great results while at the same time reducing the risk of injuries. To do so, always begin your interval workouts gradually and increase the intensity and frequency with time. Avoid pushing your body beyond limit but instead scatter your HIIT sessions across the week. You can start with short HIIT sessions involving 3 or 4 intervals of 30 seconds with recovery intervals in-between. Increase the intervals and intensity as you get more comfortable. Always begin with a warm up session.

Choose exercises you enjoy most

You want to stick to your HIIT workout plan and this can only happen if you choose fun and enjoyable exercises. If you are not the kind that loves running, then you will need to avoid including running intervals in your training. However, always make sure that your HIIT exercise of choice is engaging enough and involves the use of your larger muscle groups such as legs and arms to help increase your heart rate. Also, choose an exercise that allows you to accelerate rapidly within seconds and decelerate equally fast.

Fuel up properly

Don't try to do your HIIT workout routines on an empty stomach. To achieve the best results, you will need to supply your body with the right diet including fast-digesting carbohydrates (at minimum though) and proteins. These will fuel the muscles while at the same time providing them with the necessary amino acids needed for energy and rebuilding. Keep fats to the minimum and drink a lot of water for proper hydration.

Don't push your body too much

Have some rest days in the course of the week and don't push the body too much if it doesn't feel like doing the HIIT sessions for that particular day. During such days, go for low intensity workouts to help in the recovery process in readiness for the intense workouts the following day. If you are a beginner, go for one or two HIIT sessions per week and build up on that. As your body adapts, it will be easier to increase the intensity and intervals.

Chapter 5: Introduction To The Hiit Regimen

In the world today where beauty is put at a premium, keeping fit has become a must and an activity that takes up a lot of your time. More and more exercise regimens and diet plans are invented and are sold to those who are willing to listen to the (sometimes fallacious) scientific facts that are believed to belie their efficiency.

However, despite all these options available, the everyday man still looks for something more. Most routines are either too tough or too time consuming for someone who works the regular 9-5 shift to invest in. Expensive equipment may sometimes be a necessity as well. Instead of all these, we are all looking for something that can help us keep fit while at the same time still giving us enough time to spend for ourselves and for our affairs.

Many people are aware that the reason certain exercises are so effective is because they are capable of burning more calories than we take in on a daily basis. However, the more rigorous the workout, the more likely we are to break away from it as a habit. Also, many people take on the pain of having to memorize certain sequences of exercises simply to get their pulses up. This is not the ideal and still more reasons why many people are staying away from the fit lifestyle.

Enter the High-Intensity Interval Training regimen, also known as HIIT. This exercise routine, which has taken the fitness world by storm since its inception in the 90s, is a revolutionary system that sports the following advantages over many of the existing workout routines:

Efficiency. HIIT (High Intensity Interval Training) is an ideal exercise regimen even for the worker who is busy with his schedule. Even if one wishes to squeeze in a fat-burning session at lunch time, of if he wants to quickly lose all those extra pounds after suddenly remembering a trip to the beach he forgot was coming, HIIT can help in no way other routines can.

Many research publications have shown that only 15 minutes of interval training done 3 times a week would bring you more rewarding progress than doing the treadmills for an hour, three times a week. Also, only 2 weeks of consistent HIIT workouts can give you as much improvement in aerobic capacity as 6-8 weeks of endurance routines.

How is this possible? Many dissidents would site that three quarters of an hour on a treadmill can burn 400 calories, while 15 minutes of high-intensity workouts can only burn around 250. How can HIIT be superior?

The secret is in a process called EPOC, or Excess Post-Exercise Oxygen Consumption. This is also colloquially called the "After burn Effect". While more calories from fat are burned while exercising, HIIT pays attention to what is burned after. After burn is basically a process relating to an increased intake of oxygen as the body attempts to correct the "oxygen debt" caused by the routine. The harsher and more intense the exercise, the greater the oxygen debt is. To restore the body to a resting state, the body attempts to increase the oxygen consumption.

While this happens, the body performs several chemical processes. This includes the restoration of hormonal imbalances, replenishing those lost phosphates stores, oxidizing the built-up lactic acid to prevent cramping, and carrying out repairs of damaged cells. Because of these, energy from fatty acids is borrowed - the body breaks down the stores of fat, releasing these fatty acids into the bloodstream. These are then used by the cells as energy for the functions required in putting the body back to a resting state.

Longer and slower low-intensity cardiovascular exercises are more likely to produce a slow EPOC effect, lasting at most only a couple of hours after one works out. In the example given above, the 400 calories burned will be technically all there is, as the after burn is mostly negligible.

But sports scientists have found out that after an HIIT session, the after burn can last up to 38 hours! That's more than a day of fat burning even after you end the workout. The more intense the routine, the more energy is needed in the after burn.

Healthier Heart. Many people, even those who workout consistently, are not really used to pushing the body to its limits. The anaerobic zone, when you breach that barrier of common activity and your heart tries to jump out of your ribcage (and you feel like you can't breathe), is a place widely unknown. But it has its undeniable advantages. A certain study conducted in 2006 has mentioned that after 8 full weeks of HIIT, the participants could bike for twice longer that they could ever before, while still at the same pace. HIIT can produce extreme cardiovascular improvements.

Expense less. Aside from running, most exercise fans take the time to bike, row, jump rope, and more. And if they can't bike using a real bike or row on a real boat, they go to the gym and pay a monthly subscription just to do it. HIIT, on the other hand, does not require any equipment at all. Plyometric exercises that include jumping lunges, high knees, and more can work wonders in kicking your heart rate up fast. In fact, common exercise equipment such as dumbbells can actually lessen HIIT's efficiency due to it tendency to shift your focus to working on your muscles, instead of on your heart.

Battle Muscle Loss. Aside from exercise, people also use dieting as a means to stay fit. However, anyone who has gone down this path knows that muscle is lost along with fat. Even worse, steady-state cardiovascular routines can actually encourage the loss of these muscles.

Experts have shown that aside from weight-training, HIIT helps to preserve those muscles while burning only the fat.

Increase Overall Metabolism. Aside from having increased levels of fat burning and the preservation of existing muscles, the production of human growth hormones (HGH) can also be stimulated by HITT. In fact, studies have shown that the hormone can be upped by as much as 450% during the first day after one works out!

The human growth hormone is responsible for increasing the rate at which our body burns calories, as well as helpful in slowing down the aging process. This makes you look younger, inside out!

Unparalleled Convenience. HIIT is a routine that can be performed literally anywhere. It can be done at home in your living room, or at a cramped space in your basement. It can also be done at work, even inside a maintenance closet, for that matter (though we don't recommend it)! The concept behind the routine is so simple - simply push yourself and exert maximum effort in a heart-pumping activity for a short period, and follow it up by a short recovery period. Then repeat. No matter what time or space constraints befall you, this exercise can be done.

Unparalleled Challenge. This is not that type of exercise where you can spare some effort to chat on the phone while doing reps. Because the entire regimen is so short, you need to be working hard the whole time. But this format also offers even seasoned exercisers a different and new challenge, while also providing the newbies a chance to see quicker results.

Helps Make an Athlete Out of You! HITT has also been scientifically shown to help improve one's athletic performance. Though it does not really do much to help you bat every ball or shoot every hoop, it allows one to get the bodily endurance needed to train in these aspects.

HIIT also helps those whose athletic prowess had already been established. One problem with conventional training methods is that they provide little opportunities for well-trained athletes to improve their game. Even an increase in the volume of exercise may yield little to no improvements. However, a 2009 study had shown definitive proof that endurance and performance of even seasoned athletes can be improved by HIIT. After only 7 interval training sessions, a 2% improvement was already marked.

Helps the Ill. Cardiovascular diseases and diabetes are two of the most commonplace conditions across the world caused by a portion of the body that may be malfunctioning. In fact, those who suffer these conditions can be greatly affected by HIIT.

A 2011 study has proved that HIIT can significantly and efficiently reduce the markers of cardiovascular diseases in adolescents. This makes it a useful tool to prevent the onset of these diseases from the outset.

Also, HIIT has been shown to lower insulin resistance and cause skeletal muscle adaptations that improves glucose tolerance, aiding greatly in the case of diabetics. As much as 24% increase in insulin sensitivity has been demonstrated in studies, after only 4 weeks of HIIT workouts.

Improves the Mind. The Montreal Heart Institute found another significant (and for some, unprecedented) advantage to doing HIIT workouts. Subjects that had been performing the routine twice a week of four months actually showed a significant increase in scores from cognition tests. Brain oxygenation levels were also increased.

HIIT Procedures

As mentioned before, the regimen of HIIT is very simple. One only has to pump his heart rate to the maximum possible for a short period of time (without incurring any damage, of course).

Ideally, a session will start off with a warm up exercise, with three to ten reps of high-intensity routines right after. These routines are separated with a slower pace of medium exercise for recovery. It ends with a cool-down exercise.

The high-intensity part is ideally done at near-maximum capacity (again, that talk of pushing the limits of the body). The medium-intensity workout, on the other hand, has to be done at around 50% of the previous routine. The length and number of reps would be depending on the type of exercise being performed, but there may be as little as three reps with only twenty seconds each of intense workouts.

As for a formula, no specific one exists in the realm of HIIT, unlike in other regimens. This simply depends on the level of a person's cardiovascular development. The moderate-intensity exercises can even be as slow as simply walking. A common combination, though, would be to have a 2:1 ratio of the workout to the recovery periods. As an example, a 30-40 second workout consisting of hard sprints can be alternated with 15-20 seconds of simple jog or walk.

An entire session may also vary in terms of time. It can last any time between 4 and 30 minutes, giving rise to its popularity as the choice regimen for those who have limited time to spare.

Wait... What is "High-Intensity", Anyway?

Try doing a simple trial run of a round of the chosen workout at your most explosive pace. This will allow you to try and find out how many repetitions for one interval would suit your ability. Try beating that number or coming as close as possible to it at each round. This will make sure that you are making an effort to push yourself and outrun what you previously set.

One good way to keep track of your time and the number of rounds you were able to complete (because it hurts to keep counting while pushing yourself to the limits) is to either buy an interval clock or to download an interval app for your smartphone. This timer will help you by beeping or buzzing at the end of each programmed interval, signifying that it is time to crank your intensity down or back up.

If a person can complete 30 minutes of HIIT and still feel like he can take a relaxing stroll right after, then that person is not doing it right.

Chapter 6: Applying Hiit To Your Cardio

You can start by applying HIIT to your cardio. If you have a treadmill or a stationary bike at home, you can start doing HIIT routines today.

Treadmill HIIT Routine

Warm Up:

You should do a 2-3 mile per hour walk until you begin to sweat.

Circuit

- Start slow:

Level 2 intensity: Walk at a 2.5 mile per hour pace with a 6 incline on the treadmill. You should do this for 1 minute and 30 seconds.

- Increase the pace:

Level 4 intensity: You should run at a 6 mph pace for 1 minute and 30 seconds at a 4 incline on the treadmill.

- Ease the tension in your knees:

Level 2 intensity: Walk for 1 minute and 30 seconds at a 3 mile per hour pace. Set the incline back to 0 to give your knees a break.

- Mix it up:

Level 4 intensity: You should work with a jump rope for 1 minute to end the circuit. Do it as fast as you can. This will rest your calf muscles and your heels for the next round but it will keep your heart pounding.

You may take a 2-minute break at the end of the circuit. After 2 minutes, you should start over with the circuit. You should repeat the circuit 4 times. A beginner should be able to finish 4 rounds of this circuit in than less 30 minutes.

HIIT while Biking

You can also apply HIIT while biking. You can do this protocol in your stationary bike or in the open road.

Warm up:

Warm up at a comfortable pace for 7 minutes or until you are comfortable enough to start.

Routine:

Bike slowly for 20 seconds to set the pace and to become accustomed to the resistance. If the resistance is too weak, tighten it to simulate the resistance of the tire's contact to the open road.

Sprint for another 20 seconds. Just go as fast as you can. The speed of the sprint depends on how experienced you are at biking. Buking purists can sprint for 4-5 minutes without getting tired. Beginners will tire out within a minute. Bike slowly in the next 10 seconds

Repeat the sprint-slow cycle (steps 2 and 3) for 8 rounds. You should be done in around 4 minutes and 20 seconds. After 8 rounds, you should start biking at a comfortable pace to cooldown.

Chapter 7: Steps That Will Make Your Hiit Effective

The HIIT exercises will work best on ensuring you achieve the body you desire. But there are important steps that go hand in hand with the HIIT exercises and one should ensure that apart from exercising they ensure that they put them into practice. These steps are basic and are of essence for you to easily and quickly achieve a healthy and fit body.

Proper Nutrition

Health, fitness and nutrition are dependent on each other. To ensure your body is perfect and fit it has to be exercised, relaxed and also fed well. Diet is important as it helps you maintain a healthy weight and reduce the risk of chronic diseases. One has to ensure they have a balanced meal everyday. Ensure you have carbohydrates, proteins, vitamins and fats. To lose weight it doesn't mean you don't eat enough food. It means eating the right foods in the right quantity. Proper nutrition is of essence because of the following reasons.

1.) It ensures proper growth and development as it provides you with the raw materials which your cells are made of.

2.) It is important for muscle tissue building and development. It is through proper nutrition that you enhance the growth of lean muscle tissue and its maintenance.

3.) It is the best way for disease prevention. With a balanced nutrition one should ensure that the foods are rich in vitamins, minerals and anti oxidants.

4.) It is also essential for immune system support. Fruits and vegetables are very important for your immune system.

5.) It is through proper nutrition that one boosts their body energy.

Body Relaxation

Relaxation isn't about you sitting and watching television the whole day. There are other important forms of body relaxation that one can practice which will help in maintaining their general health e.g. meditation, yoga etc. Relaxation helps in body building as it reduces stress and this helps you to maintain a good body health and will allow exercising efficiently. Through relaxation we aim at relaxing the major muscle groups in our body and thus help you feel refreshed.

Relaxation will help you in the following ways:

• Slowing our heart rate

• Lowering blood pressure

• Increasing blood flow to major muscles

• Reducing muscle tension and chronic pain

• Lowering fatigue

Proper Hydration

It is always very important for one to be well hydrated before, during and after exercising. This is important because water helps in regulating body temperature, lubricating joints and also help in transporting nutrients through the body thus allows you to have enough energy and also good health. The signs of dehydration are as highlighted below:

• Dizziness

• Nausea

• Muscle cramps

• Dry mouth

• You stop sweating

• Heart palpitations

Dehydration decreases your performance during exercising. This is because one tends to sweat a lot and water is lost in the process. This is therefore the reason why we insist on proper hydration which will help you have an effective training session.

Resting And Sleeping Enough

It is very important for you to rest and sleep well, especially after HIIT exercises. Sleeping keeps your mind and body healthy. Through sleeping you will relax your muscles and also recover your lost energy. Getting enough rest and sleep will help you function well the whole day, allowing you to exercise your HIIT program with ease.

Chapter 8: Strategic Supplementation

I've found that a few supplements help minimize hunger or fatigue that some may experience while fasting. The supplements I recommend in this program include:

Fiber (psyllium or methylcellulose). The recommended dose is 3 to 5 grams twice daily. Fiber increases sensations of fullness and studies show that it decreases hunger.[29]

Healthy fats. Healthy fats include omega-3 fatty acids and medium-chain triglycerides. For omega-3 fatty acids, the recommended dose is 2 to 4 grams twice daily. For medium-chain triglycerides (as MCT oil or coconut oil), the recommended dose is 5 to 10 grams twice daily. Studies show that the anti-inflammatory effects of the omega-3s may help with weight loss. [30] Medium-chain triglycerides suppress the accumulation of body fat, according to other studies[31].

Branched-chain amino acids. A dose of 5 grams twice daily is helpful for reducing hunger pangs and preventing muscle breakdown associated with restrictive dieting and intense exercise.[32] Branched-chain amino acids stabilize blood glucose and prevent carbohydrate cravings that some may experience on their fasting days.[33]

Creatine. (Optional) A dose of 3 to 5 mg of creatine daily helps supply muscle tissue with energy demands required for brief, vigorous exercise bouts. Creatine is helpful for those engaged in resistance-based, high-intensity exercise.

When is the best time to take these supplements? I suggest taking the supplements on a regular schedule, regardless of whether you are feeding or fasting. Many find that taking supplements twice daily, once in the morning and once in the evening, works best.

Fiber

The average American diet lacks sufficient fiber. For healthy adult males, the daily recommended fiber intake is about thirty grams each day, but actual consumption is closer to 10 to 12 grams. That's unfortunate because fiber contributes to feelings of fullness, stabilizes blood sugar, and helps to reduce blood cholesterol.

Fiber slows the absorption of carbohydrate from the gut into the bloodstream, and thus prevents rapid surges in blood glucose that might otherwise trigger the release of the fat storage hormone, insulin.

Recommended sources of fiber include psyllium husk or methylcellulose at a dose of three to five grams twice daily.

Healthy Fats

Healthy fats are another important supplement to consider while following a program of intermittent fasting and high-intensity interval training.

Healthy fats accentuate the benefits of intermittent fasting by increasing the production of ketone bodies, which are used as an alternative energy source by the brain and muscle tissue. Fats also reduce hunger and improve cognition, according to some studies.[34]

Fish oil capsules and bottled fish oil are the sources of omega-3 that I recommend. While capsules are easier for travel, I recommend taking a high-quality liquid form to avoid taking large amounts of the inert gelatin that make up the capsules. One teaspoon of a high-quality fish oil contains about two grams of omega-3s. I recommend taking two grams of a high-quality omega-3 twice daily. If you are on anti-coagulant therapy, be sure to check with your physician before taking omega-3s, as they can potentiate the blood-thinning effects of medications such as aspirin and warfarin.

The amount of medium-chain triglycerides (MCTs) I recommend is ten grams (approximately one tablespoon) twice daily. The easiest way to take MCTs is in the form of coconut oil, which you can find in the cooking oil section of most supermarkets. A convenient way to take coconut oil is to mix one tablespoon into your morning coffee or tea.

One precaution: Don't increase your dose of these oils too quickly. Doing so can lead to gastrointestinal distress and diarrhea. Start with about 1/2 to one teaspoon and increase the oils as tolerated to the recommended doses above.

Branched-Chain Amino Acids

The branched-chain amino acids (leucine, isoleucine, and valine) are unique among the twenty or so amino acids used by the body. They become particularly important when glucose, our main energy source, runs low because the body uses the branched-chain amino acids as an alternative energy source. Humans can't synthesize these and other essential amino acids, but they play a key role in energy metabolism.

The branched-chain amino acids also promote weight loss by increasing signals to the brain that indicate fullness or satiety.[35] Other studies find that they increase fat oxidation, the rate at which our bodies use fat as an energy source.[36]

The recommended dose is ten grams mixed with 8 to 12 ounces of water. The branched-chain amino acids are available in powdered form. You can find them at most health food stores.

During periods of intermittent fasting and high-intensity interval training, I recommend taking five grams of branched-chain amino acids mixed with carbonated water (to improve mixing and decrease their bitter taste). Do this immediately before and after exercising.

Creatine

Creatine plays a key role in maintaining energy stores for fast-contracting muscle. When you begin a high-intensity interval training program such as the one described here, the main source of energy for contracting muscle comes from the breakdown of creatine to form adenosine triphosphate (ATP). Approximately 95% of the body's total creatine is located in skeletal muscle, and intense exercise rapidly depletes creatine stores.[37] Other pathways produce energy for muscle contraction lasting longer than about 10 seconds, but the creatine phosphate system is the most important. For this reason, I recommend 3 to 5 grams of creatine daily while performing high-intensity interval training.

Chapter 9: Hiit With Bodyweight Workouts

It is apparent that the first two programs are better performed with the aid of machines, but if having or looking for one does not suit your lifestyle, then this will definitely work for you. There is entirely no need for you to invest on any equipment or gym membership. As long as there's adequate space on your home to exercise, losing weight is just a matter of work.

There are over fifty different bodyweight exercises and you can mix these up to create a full body workout routine. Aside from losing weight, you are sure to get a well-toned body. Equal distribution of work on different muscle groups will keep the development balanced. Therefore, if workouts are done properly, and schedules are kept strictly, you'll have that Hollywood-worthy body.

Training Guide

This is the foundation of almost all exercises. If you are looking to lose weight with the bodyweight HIIT program, expect to gain strength and improve endurance on the side.

Compared to running and cycling, bodyweight exercises are more difficult despite its convenience. Different muscle groups will move at the same time, hence requiring more effort and concentration.

Level 1 : Tabata Method

Level one of this program may shock most beginners. There is no way to lower the intensity of these exercises but to lessen sets, or increase time limits.

Begin with an intimate warm-up by jogging in place, or doing high-knee exercises. Afterwards, box the following exercises to sets of 30 seconds, consisting of 20 seconds of work, and 10 seconds of stationary rest.

8 sets of Jump Squats

8 sets of Pushups

8 sets of Planks

8 sets of Sit-ups

8 sets of Burpees

Complete every set of every exercise and you'll get a total exercise time of 24 minutes. Maintain this routine for two weeks.

This may seem intimidating, but this is level one. What made this routine easy is that there's no pressure in accomplishing specific repetitions. You are allowed to do as much as you can for 20 seconds. Once you begin to progress, however, strive to beat your previous record. A journal will come in handy if you are entirely serious with this.

Level 2 : 24-Minute Classics

The intensity of this routine will be focused on stamina for you will engage in continuous movement for 6 long minutes.

Warm-up with high-knee exercises. Raise your knees to your hips to get your heart rate up. You can follow this up with high-knee slow jogs, or high-knee jogs if your heart rate isn't going up fast enough. Do this for five minutes, and then follow this exercise sequence:

10 Burpees

20 Alternating Lunges

20 Squats

10 Diver's Pushups

Do these exercises continuously for 6 minutes. Repeat as many rounds as you can within the time limit, then follow it up with a 2-minute rest. Start from the top and finish a total of 3 rounds.

Ideally, this workout is maintained for three weeks. However, as you progress, higher intensity must be gradually added. Increase repetitions, or beat your previous record with higher number of rounds accomplished in 6 minutes.

Level 3 : Muscle Burn Workout

This is where things get serious. You will have to push yourself more to survive the final leg of the bodyweight exercises HIIT program because your muscles will surely burn.

After the similar warm-up with level two, you will perform the following exercises. There is no time limit, but take note of the repetitions. Take a 30 second rest between each exercise.

40 Jump Squats

30 Pushups

50 Sit-ups

10 Tricep Dips

20 Split Jumps

30 Second Burpees

You don't have to repeat anything. Once you finish the burpee, you are done for the day. If everything is a little too much, decrease the number of repetitions, or take longer rests. Keep this exercise for two weeks.

Training Schedule

It is highly recommended that you do not skip level one even if you're not a beginner. This will help you measure your capabilities better, and prepare you accordingly for the program's progression. Each level is open for tweaking, so if you find it lacking, you are free to increase repetitions or decrease times. What's important is for you to adhere to the schedule.

	Mon	Tue	Wed	Thu	Fri	Sat	Sun
W	Level	R	Level	R	Level	R	Stre

ee k 1	1	es t	1	es t	1	es t	tch
W ee k 2	Level 1 Incre ased Reps	R es t	Level 1 Incre ased Reps	R es t	Level 1 Incre ased Reps	R es t	Stre tch
W ee k 3	Level 2	R es t	Level 2	R es t	Level 2	R es t	Stre tch
W ee k 4	Level 2 Incre ased round	R es t	Level 2 Incre ased round	R es t	Level 2 Incre ased round	R es t	Stre tch

	s		s		s		
Week 5	Level 2 Increased rounds	Rest	Level 2 Increased rounds	Rest	Level 2 Increased rounds	Rest	Stretch
Week 6	Level 3	Rest	Level 3	Rest	Level 3	Rest	Stretch
Week 7	Level 3 Decreased	Rest	Level 3 Decreased	Rest	Level 3 Decreased	Rest	Stretch

	time		time		time		

Reminders

The reminders in the first two program applies to this as well. There are, however, additional points that you may overlook when performing the exercises.

Effective workouts aren't measured by high number of repetitions, but by perfection of form. Therefore, be mindful of your body when doing bodyweight exercises. Squats, for example, require you to keep your back straight all throughout the exercise.

Stretches won't be limited to your lower body this time. There will be tension in your arms, back and core, because of planks, burpees and push-ups, so make sure to give these muscle groups proper stretching.

Chapter 10: Advanced High Intensity Interval Training

Advanced HIIT at home

Taking high intensity interval training to the highest level means you really want to challenge yourself seriously. Advanced HIIT intends to push you to your greatest ability in a very short time period with Cardio exercises.

The following is a series of exercises for an Advanced HIIT session.

Squat Jacks

Stand up with feet close together. Hold the weight about chin level. Then, squat. Tighten your ABS and squeeze the ball to engage the muscles. Jump and spread your feet while keeping yourself low. Go back to the squat position and repeat the instruction for 30 seconds or 30 repetitions.

Star Jumps

Do this on grass or mat. Slightly bend your knees. Spread your feet with shoulder-width on a flat surface. Jump as high as you can. While in the air, fully extend your arms and legs out to your side. It would form a star shape with your body. Bring your arms and legs inward near your body as you to start to fall. Bend your knees when you land on the ground. Then, squat and push off upright again. Repeat the procedure.

Mt. Climbers

Assume a push-up position with your arms stretch forward. Keep your body straight from your head to your ankles. While your lower back is arched, raise your right knee toward your chest. Hold this position for a few seconds before you return to the starting position. Repeat the steps with the other leg.

Thigh Slap Push Ups

Do the push up position with your arms stretched. Drop down to the ground while you bring your knees forward. Then, slap your hands against the thighs. Go back to the push up position and repeat the procedure.

Squats with Front Leg Slide

Press your back against the wall. Place your feet slightly out in front of you. Then, raise your right leg a few inches off the floor. Squat until your weighted knee reaches a 90 degree bend. Hold this position for a few seconds before pushing yourself up and back against the wall. Repeat the steps with the other leg.

Jumping Lunges

Start with one leg in the front. It should be at a 90 degree in the squat position and back leg behind you. Lower your body and jump. Switch your feet in the air by moving back leg in front and the front leg in back. In reverse legs, go straight into a lunge. Do the entire drill while keeping your chest and torso upright.

Begin your advanced HIIT workout with these simple exercises. Yes, these are not so easy to do. But if you become familiar with the exercises, it will be easier for you. Practice makes perfect.

Outdoor exercises

You need to have a regular exercise to enhance your strength, speed, endurance and physical endurance. Using treadmill and other equipment is fine, but why don't you try doing it outside? While you work out, you'll see different views, meet different people and have a chance to breathe fresh air. You can also keep yourself from distractions and unnecessary activities. Plus, you can do it with your friends or partner.

So what are you waiting for? Wear your running shoes and try these outdoor exercises.

Hill sprints

You need to sprint up the hill and walk down the hill. It seemed simple to do, but it's not. Your heart will beat faster and you will feel your legs burning while sprinting up for several times.

There are some tips you have to keep in mind when doing this. You need to chin up and keep your eyes forward. Never look down no matter how tired you are. As you sprint up, your chest should be out and shoulders back. Clenching your fists isn't necessary. Lightly squeeze your fists or run with your palms open.

Keeping your arms bent at a 90-degree angle is another thing to do. Move them up and down as you run. But don't let your arms cross over your body while sprinting. Also, you need to pick your knees up high and keep your hips forward. Don't move from side to side.

Football field sprints

Of course, you need to go to football fields to do this exercise. If you can't find one, look for alternative like a very wide vacant place or oval field. Sprint 40 yards, and then walk 60 yards. You can repeat it as long as you can.

Sled pulls or pushes

If you get tired of running, you still have something to do outside your home. Get a sled. Push or pull it for 30 seconds. Have an active rest for 30 seconds and repeat pulling or pushing the sled as long as you can. You can even try to push a car if you want.

Running bleachers

A simple running rapidly increases our heart rate. Running bleachers is more difficult than that. Your heart rate will increase up into the training zone because it is more intense. Its effect is similar to the intense exercises you do at home. You also need to have an active rest after sprinting up. Go down by walking.

Since it's not an easy exercise, be ready and concentrate. You need to pay attention to your form and focus on each and every step to avoid accident. Be careful because you might have broken bones if you stumble and fall.

Sprints in the park

This is the simplest form of running. Go outside your house and start running for your desired time. Rest for 30 seconds and start running again. Repeat for several times.

Jump rope

Have a jumping rope and start jumping for 25 seconds. Have a break for 15 seconds and jump again. It's just a simple activity. If you know how to jump at the right time, it will not be difficult for you.

There are a lot of things you can do outside your home. But you need to focus and be careful to avoid accidents.

Chapter 11: Hiit For Endurance

To build endurance, you don't have to spend hours of your daily life training and doing intense exercises. HIIT is a great way for building endurance since it focuses on the major endurance-building points in the body.

One of the main elements of endurance is cardiovascular performance. This refers to the way your heart works and the subsequent working of the circulatory system in response to heart's pumping. The functioning of the heart can be measured by three determinants.

Heart Rate

This is the rate of your heart beating per minute. The more your heart beats in a minute, the more blood is pumped to the body and the faster your body moves towards endurance.

Stroke Volume

This refers to the blood amount that is pumped every time the heart beats. Since there is a direct relationship between the stroke volume and endurance, a higher stroke volume is beneficial for the body.

Contractility

This refers to the force with which your heart pumps blood to the body. The stronger the force, the farther the blood travels. If contractility is higher, an individual has more blood flowing to the exercising muscles. This blood is laden with oxygen and nutrients that are then utilized by the skeletal muscles for strength and repair.

113

How Is Endurance Built?

Endurance is not only a measurement of how hard your heart is pumping blood. It also refers to the amount of oxygen that can be delivered to your muscles. This variable is called VO2. This variable depends on the factors mentioned above as well as on the amount of oxygen that is extracted from the blood that enters the muscles. Not all the oxygen that is taken to the muscles by the blood is taken by the muscles. The oxygen has to be extracted first and the more oxygen extraction capacity the muscles have, more oxygen they will receive.

Another factor that contributes to endurance is the mitochondrial density. It is common knowledge that mitochondria is the power house of the cell. What this means is that it is involved in the production of energy in the form of ATP.

This energy is produced through different cycles that take place in the mitochondria. The higher the mitochondrial density, the more energy is produced for the consumption of the body.

How Does HIIT Build Endurance?

HIIT builds endurance by working on all the variables that are mentioned above. It enhances the stroke volume for ensuring a greater amount of blood flow to the skeletal muscles. Moreover, it also has an effect on contractility and increases the pumping force of the heart.

As far as mitochondrial density is concerned, HIIT is a great alternative to aerobic exercises for increasing your mitochondrial density. If there are more mitochondria is the body, more energy production takes place and that gives the muscles more endurance.

Another way in which HIIT induces endurance is by increasing the number of enzymes present in the mitochondria. As mentioned above, energy is produced in the mitochondria through different cycles. In all the steps of these cycles, different enzymes act on the substrate to form a product. These enzymes have their distinctive activities that are essential for energy production. HIIT leads to an increase in these enzymes and these enzymes then further increase the endurance in skeletal muscles.

When you perform HIIT, it shifts the signalling pathway in the body from a slower to a faster one. For breakdown of nutrients and extraction of energy from them, the mitochondria are activated through a 'switch' in the body called PGCa. During high intensity exercises, the signalling pathway for activation of this switch is a lot faster. As a result of that, the enzymes' activity is enhanced and the mitochondrial density is also increased.

HIIT and VO2

As mentioned above, the VO2 levels in the blood determine how much oxygen is getting to the skeletal muscles and other parts of the body. HIIT has shown to significantly enhance VO2 levels in the body and enhances stroke volume. Since the stroke volume is enhanced through high intensity workouts, more blood gets sent to the body every single time the heart contracts. This is a good thing for the skeletal muscles since they start getting more blood.

The circulatory system of the body is responsible for transport of nutrients and oxygen to the muscles and other organs. When the skeletal muscles get more blood, they also get more oxygen and nutrients. This is essential for proper growth and functioning of the muscles.

Using this oxygen, they can respire and release energy using the mitochondria present in them. At the same time, the amino acids in the nutrients are further used for repair and for synthesis of new proteins that are needed for the muscles.

High intensity workouts also increase cardiac contractility which refers to the force with which the heart pumps blood. As the pumping force is increased, the blood reaches all muscles and organs of the body. When skeletal muscles get more blood, they build up endurance. It is due to this excessive endurance that the individual has shorter recovery time and can perform much better in gym sessions.

HIIT Builds Endurance In Skeletal Muscles

High intensity workouts also build endurance in skeletal muscles. When you perform these exercises, the vasculature of the skeletal muscle is changed. The vasculature refers to the size and number of blood vessels that are present in the area. Due to these workouts, tiny blood vessels become apparent in the skeletal muscles.

They enhance the heart stroke by sending more blood to the heart. The muscles, when contracting, send blood back to the left ventricle of the heart. If more blood is being sent to the heart, it means more blood is being oxygenated too. Thus, heart stroke is enhanced and more blood is sent back to the body in oxygenated form. This increases the amount of nutrients getting to the muscles.

HIIT also enhances endurance by increasing the strength of muscle fibres.

The muscles fibres are made up on proteins. In high intensity workouts, the blood circulation is enhanced and more of these proteins are being made using the amino acids present in the blood. This enhances the flexibility of the muscle fibres and makes them stronger.

Motor Units And HIIT

The skeletal muscle fibres have something called motor units. These units are important for signalling in the muscles and for building endurance. High intensity workouts increase the number of motor units present in the body. This can aid in two things.

• If more motor units are present in the skeletal muscles, then muscle coordination improves and the person has better endurance.

- Motor units also help to reduce the fatigue time for exercises. As such, anyone with enhanced motor units does not tend to get tired quickly.

Does HIIT Affect Qmax?

Qmax is referred to the maximum amount of blood that your heart can pump to the body in a minute. It has been seen in studies that high intensity workouts have little or no significant effect on Qmax. On the contrary, low intensity workouts such as aerobic workout plans are great for increasing Qmax.

Therefore, HIIT takes cardiovascular pathways to increase endurance. It increases the density of mitochondria in the cells along with enhancing the functioning of mitochondrial enzymes. Furthermore, it strengthens the muscle fibres by giving them more proteins for repair and strength. High intensity workouts also increase endurance by overall increasing the VO2 max and by keeping the oxygen volume in the blood high at all times, for transfer to the skeletal muscles.

Chapter 12: Incorporate Visualization In Your Life

Visualization can easily make you a winner, & if you want to become successful in your entire life, you can try visualization. A positive attitude is necessary for your success in life because it'll develop confidence & self-esteem. The positive attitude will improve your overall mood because you can easily enrich your life to reduce the effects of negative thinking on your life. Following are some useful exercises that'll help you to just develop a positive attitude:

Open your Mind

If you really want to develop a positive attitude, you should open your mind to think positively & listen to the viewpoints of other people. Understand their perspective, & respect their thoughts & accept their suggestions & criticism with such an open mind. Pay attention to their ideas & thoughts to just find endless opportunities for you.

Write Down 10 Things you're Grateful for Regularly

You've to simply write down ten things on a regular basis that you're grateful on a daily basis. It'll help you to think positively, & you can quickly develop an optimistic look. The practice will actually help you to be thankful for the good things you already have in your life. There's really no need to write only big things because the little things are sufficient to just see a change in your life.

Learn to Meditate on a Regular Basis

Meditation will actually help you to stay away from negativity, & you'll feel physically better. The meditation is equally useful even for a person who's not spiritual. You really need to find a quiet & peaceful spot to meditate. You can easily meditate in a quiet room to avoid any distraction. Focus on positive things while using different meditation techniques.

Affirmations to Develop Self-Esteem

If you really want to develop self-esteem with Affirmation, then focus on your strengths & the things that you can do well. There's no need to focus on your faults because it'll hold you back. Do not worry about failures because the failures will make you healthy. It'll basically help you to look at you in a better way. Following are some positive affirmations to develop self-esteem:

• My self-esteem is escalating on a regular basis

• I accept my defeat & focus on its positive aspects

• I've trust in my abilities

• I can do anything

• My confidence & self-esteem are high

• I can easily achieve everything as per my wish

• I love & trust myself

• I understand my abilities

• I can speak to the positive thoughts of myself

• I'm beautiful & creative

Identify Negative Thoughts & Fears to Kill Them

In the first step, you've to ask yourself; either you've negative thoughts or positive thoughts for the major part of the day. For this purpose, you're in really need to identify negative thoughts. The negative thoughts start with:

• "Cannot do" instead of "can."

• No, instead of Yes

• Not confident instead of confident

• Failure instead of success

If you're feeding these thoughts in your mind, unfortunately, you're feeding the negativity to it. The biggest problem of this era is simply captivation of the people by their thoughts. You really often let your thoughts control you, instead of controlling them for your benefits. It's crucial for you to learn control of your thoughts.

Ignored Tools to Power Your Mind

Mental strength is crucial to develop to deal with different problems & complications of your life. There're mainly five things that're often overlooked, as:

• Confidence & belief

• Ability to overcome adversity

• Ability to tolerate pain

• Desire & determination to continue your journey

• Ability to conquer fear

Confidence

Confidence is the foundation of mental strength because it can easily help you to just reach the top of any sport. You should've confidence that you've the ability to achieve your goal. If you think that you aren't capable of achieving your desired goals, it'll be your failure, & you may not be really able to move on. You should simply believe yourself because any negative influence can shatter your confidence & increase self-doubt. It's crucial to believe that you've the ability to achieve your goals.

Overcome adversity

Everyone face hardship at one time or another, & for some people, it can be really harder to bear these situations than others. You may actually find it hard to deal with injuries, family problems, & professional as well as personal commitments. You should've the ability to overcome hardships in such a convincing manner. It's crucial for you to take everything positively because adversities in your entire life can polish you. These types of situations can be really helpful to filter useless & selfish people around you. Remind yourself that you can bear these hardships & these're good for you instead of feeling hopeless.

Tolerate pain

Pain will simply come into your life in different forms, as pain from an injury, mental fatigue, broken relations, etc. You should've the ability to tolerate pain in your entire life because this can take you to a new level of success. Your success is actually often hidden behind struggle & hardships. Learn to tolerate pain, & it'll ultimately increase the strength of your mind. A strong mind will give you the courage to face every bad happening & adversity in your entire life.

Get Rid of Negative Environment

Carefully look around to just find out the people giving negative energy. There're lots of people around you who actually love to share negative things with you. It's not good to give the control of your thoughts in the hands of these people. You should simply handle everything & try to remove these people from your life. If there're special bad memories in your entire life, try to forget everything by changing your place. Try to leave all those people who actually know these things & can repeat these incidents in front of you. Try to make a distance with these people & make a new circle.

Chapter 13: Hiit F.A.Q.S

Can I be too out of shape or overweight to do HIIT?

No. Very poorly conditioned trainees will benefit tremendously with a pedalling device. If no such device is available in the home, you can do the easier exercises described previously, and manipulate intensity for compatibility with your level of fitness. Poorly fit people should initially work at an RPE of 5-7.

What about smokers?

Smokers can do HIIT, and like any other demographic, should apply HIIT rules as needed.

Can I be too old for HIIT?

No. Again, the rules apply as they do for beginners or the poorly conditioned.

Should I first get my doctor's approval?

Like the general population, many doctors don't know much about HIIT. However, your physician can order a fasting glucose test to screen for diabetes. A routine physical will also screen for high blood pressure.

If you're concerned about heart health, have a cardiologist give you a thorough exam. The existence of medical conditions usually won't contraindicate HIIT, but they can alter how you do it or how frequently you fuel your body.

For example, if your doctor discovers you have osteoporosis, you may need to avoid box jumping and lunge jumps. If you have diabetes, you can aim for RPEs of up to 10, but you must monitor your blood sugar level!

I'd rather use my home cardio equipment; what are suggestions?

Find a setting that you can do for between 15 and 30 seconds, but not 31. That's your work interval. Alternate this with easy pacing. A treadmill routine may be a fixed speed with varying inclines, a fixed incline with varying speed, or a combination. A pedalling routine may involve varying pedal resistances if the machine allows it.

If I use a treadmill, can I hold on?

During work as well as rest intervals, never hold on! This will sabotage your goals. Hold on only when changing the setting from work to rest, as by then you'll be depleted of energy and need the balance to change the controls. But other than that, and sipping water, do not hold on.

How safe is HIIT?

HIIT is relatively safe on the joints and muscles because the work intervals are so brief. However, it's not advisable for obese individuals to do box jumping, lunge jumps or other high impact manoeuvres until they lose some weight. Otherwise they're at increased risk of knee injury and possibly plantar fasciitis (heel pain).

Can I do HIIT on the same day as strength training?

No. Your body needs ample recovery opportunity with HIIT. A same-day weight lifting session will compete for the limited recovery reserves. Eating more will not solve this problem. Furthermore, the psychology of knowing you have both strength training and HIIT on the same day can be daunting to manage.

Is HIIT once a week beneficial?

Yes, but since HIIT can be completed in under 30 minutes, reserve at least one more slot per week for it. You'll get results much faster.

Can I do more than eight cycles?

A HIIT session may last 45 minutes simply because the trainee takes long recovery intervals, despite only eight or fewer work segments. However, more than 10 cycles are not necessary, and in fact, often, a noticeable declination in output occurs by the fifth or sixth work interval. If you feel you can do more than 10, even more than eight, this is a sign that your first eight were submaximal! Instead of doing more than eight, focus on making your next HIIT session more intense.

Can I follow a HIIT session with steady state training?

Yes. After completing all your cycles, you can do some low intensity, fixed-pace movement, but there's no need to go beyond 20 minutes.

If I do HIIT, should I abandon altogether steady state training?

A good recommendation is two HIIT sessions per week and one steady state. If you're game for three HIIT sessions a week, you can toss in a steady state session, but make sure none of these are on a strength training day.

Though HIIT is superior to steady state, this doesn't mean that steady state lacks virtues. Get the best of both worlds: Do HIIT primarily, and then secondary to that, steady state. But if you have three slots open per week of cardio, at least two must be HIIT. And remember, don't do any kind of cardio session on the same day as strength training.

How fast will it be before I see fat burning results?

If you combine HIIT with strength training and mindful eating, results will be fast. If you're already doing strength training and steady state, but add HIIT to the picture, you'll see faster results. If you're in a fat loss rut, HIIT will lift you out of it. You may see fat loss results within a week.

I'm already lean; can HIIT make me even leaner?

Yes. For instance, if you're a woman at 17 percent body fat and you want to drop to 14 percent, and all that long duration, steady state cardio isn't helping, then switch to HIIT and see what happens!

Must the work interval always be 30 seconds maximum?

Some trainees may benefit more with longer intervals. A prime example is a very poorly conditioned person, who can't achieve an RPE greater than 7 or even 6, due to other interfering issues such as limitations with mobility due to excess body weight. This trainee may struggle to get up a flight of stairs, for example, but can't move fast enough to invoke notable cardiorespiratory fatigue within 30 seconds.

However, if this trainee continues climbing, then as one minute approaches, so will exhaustion. This phenomenon may also occur with trying to ambulate as quickly as possible on a flat surface. Physical challenges may prevent fast-enough ambulation to wear out the trainee in only 30 seconds; to elicit marked fatigue, they must keep going, sometimes for two minutes (depending on the mode).

Recovery Intervals

Never sit or stand still for a rest interval. Even a very poorly conditioned trainee should remain on their feet and keep moving. The recovery or rest interval can consist of any kind of easy-going or casual movement. The following are examples:

* Marching (including high knee) in place

* Side-to-side marching (including high knee or knee flexion—foot behind buttocks)

* Pacing

* Box tapping (tap ball of foot, alternating feet, atop stepping-box, stool or bench)

* Light kicking motions

* Very shallow stationary lunges

* Slow staircase walking

* For cardio equipment: light walking/jogging or pedalling

Chapter 14: Eight Week Hiit Workout

This next program has been divided into two, each one four weeks. In each one, you will do exactly the same exercises but the stakes will go up.

Phase One

Weeks One Through Four

These are designed to help you get into the frame of mind needed and to get your body ready. Pull in as much intensity as you can in this phase but do keep your own personal limitations in mind. You might think it's best to really push yourself from day one but it is better to test things out first, gauge the depth as it were.

Phase Two

Weeks Five Through Eight

Now that you have a good understanding of what it's all about and your body is conditioned, it's time to work on the extra fat. Because you have already adapted through phase one, your body is going to respond quickly to the extra work you are going to throw at it so keep an eye on your figure as your shape begins to change.

In both phase one and phase two, you will follow these formats:

AMRAP – as many reps as you can of the moves in a set amount of time, determined up front – normally 10 or 20 minutes. This will keep your focus on the maximum work in the minimum amount of time while giving you benchmarks for progress. For week one, for example, you log how many rounds or reps you have

143

down in total and in week two, you will try to do better than that.

Ladders – this is a descending repetition that starts you at a high rate of intensity and ends at the same rate. You focus on doing all the work efficiently, with maximum efforts to kickstart the most effective metabolic response

Strength Circuits – when you move between exercises quickly, your body doesn't get the chance to recover fully so you are adding in cardio work to increase the calorie burn. To ensure you activate the fast twitching muscle fibers, you should choose loads that are a little heavier than usual.

Day One: AMRAP (Full Body)

Sled Push

Load up a sled in a wide-open space and grip the posts high up keeping your arms straight. Push forwards deliberately, using your knees to drive you forward and keeping your hips as low as you can until you have moved the set distances. Turn and get ready to go in the opposite direction for the next round.

Dumbbell Thruster

Stand, place your feet about shoulder-width apart and turn out your toes. Hold a dumbbell in each hand at shoulder height, keeping your elbows turned down. Kick back your hips and go down deep into a squat. Extend your hips and legs and stand up very quickly, using that momentum to push up the weights above your head until your arms are extended fully. Bring the weights back down to your shoulders and repeat straight away.

Dumbbell Renegade Row

Go into a plank position resting your hands on dumbbells that are under your shoulders and parallel to the floor. Maintain a straight line with your hips, head, and heels and keep your hips square. Alternate rows with the dumbbells, bringing them to your ribs, keeping your elbows close in and head in a neutral position.

Dumbbell Walking Lunge

Holding a dumbbell in each hand, down at your sides, step forward into a lunge. Bend both of the knees and lower down to the floor, with your knee over the edge of your toes. Using your trailing foot, push off and extend your legs out. Bring the trailing leg to the front and go straight into another lunge. Repeat on alternative legs.

Days Two and Four – Active Recovery

When you first start, you are going to want to do this as much as you can to get rid of the fat but that is a big mistake. You should have at least two active recovery days every week, in between training days. Doing some mild activities can get your blood flowing properly, and move vital nutrients into the cells and the waste out. This will push your progress forward and you will even burn a few calories in the process. Some good examples of activities to do on your rest days are:

Do these at a pace that is easy to moderate and for between 30 and 60 minutes:

Bike Riding

Canoeing

Hiking

Paddle boarding

Pilates

Swimming

Tai Chi

Walking

Yoga

Day Three: Strength & Conditioning Ladders

Push-Ups

Lie on the floor with your legs extended backward and your hands flat on the floor just over shoulder-width apart keeping your heels, hips, and head in a line. Stiffen your body and lower your chest slowly until your elbows are at an angle of 90 degrees. Push forcibly back up to the start.

Goblet Squats

Stand straight with your feet placed shoulder-width apart and hold one dumbbell to your chest. Your elbows should be down and your chest lifted up. Bending the knees, squat to at least parallel, lower if you can, and then push up, using your heels, back to standing.

Assisted Pull-Ups

Loop a super band around a pull-up bar and stand on a box. Grip the bar overhand and then place one foot into the band Step completely off the box so you are hanging from the bar. Contracting the shoulder blades, push your elbows down and then back so that your chest rises up to the bar. Pause and then return to your starting position

Burpees

From a standing position, crouch and put your hands on the floor. Jump, pushing your legs back, into a plank. Do one push-u-, bring your feet back beneath you and then stand up and jump as high as you can with your hands stretched above you. Land and go straight into a crouch and repeat.

Medicine-Ball Slam

Grip a medicine ball in front of you using both hands. Using one movement, lift it above your head, stretching your arms up as far as you can and come up onto the toes. Slam the ball down using your entire body, drop your hips, contract those abs and slam that ball to the ground. Pick up and repeat immediately.

Day Five: Strength Circuits & HIIT

Barbell Deadlift

Stand with a barbell in front of you. Your feet should be at hips width apart and your toes under the bar. Keep your back flat and push your hips back; bend the knees until you can get hold of the bar in alternating grip outside of the legs. Brace to your core, bring the shoulder blades in and then stand, bringing the bar up in a line along your body until it is fully extended. Return slowly back to the starting position, touch briefly down and repeat.

Dumbbell Bench Press

Grip a dumbbell in each hand and stretch your arms straight out over your chest. Your palms should be facing away. Bend the elbows and drop the weights slowly down until your arms are at an angle of 90 degrees and your elbows and shoulders are lined up. Extend the arms out forcefully to the start and, at the top, squeeze your chest.

Farmer's Carry

Hold a set of kettlebells or heavy dumbbells down at your sides, shoulders retracted. Step forward in small steps keeping the knees bent slightly to stop the weights from swinging; walk fast until you have covered the set distance

Airdyne Bike

Set the Airdyne to a moderate tension and then pedal as hard as you can, pulling as hard as you can, fast. Do this for the set time, and then remove your feet from the pedals and your hands from the handles until your rest period is over.

Rowing Machine

Make sure the foot strap is comfortable across the instep and grip the handles overhand. Plant your heels, straighten your back and arms and push back using your legs as far as you can. Now pull the handle towards your chest, pushing your elbows behind and leaning backward from the hips. Reverse and return to your start position.

Inverted Row

Put a barbell on a rack at the thigh or lower height. Grip the bar underhand with your hands shoulder-width apart and stretch your legs. Lift up the hips, brace and pull yourself into a straight line. Push the elbows back, pull your arms into your sides and keep your body rigid then pull up. Lower back down and repeat immediately.

Create Your Own HIIT Plan

HIIT workouts are so effective that you will want to carry on and, while you can choose from thousands of tailored plans, sometimes you might want to create your own. Here's how to do it:

Length

A HIIT workout can form a few minutes up to a whole hour. Pick the time length that suits you but, if you intend to go over half an hour, mix in some low intensity exercises as well.

Intervals

Because HIIT is based on exercising at your maximal effort for the shortest time, with brief rest periods thrown in, you can set your time intervals for between 20 and 60 seconds. Do be sensible about this. It might sound easy to do burpees for one minute, believe me, that is going to feel like an incredibly long time when you are working at maximum effort. Think about that when you set your intervals. You could follow the Tabata rules of 20

154

seconds followed by 10 seconds of rest, repeated 8 times. Then you rest for 60 seconds.

Moves

This is the best bit, choosing the exercises you want to do. Pick your favorites and put them all together Mix it up, and make it fun.

Chapter 15: Your 30 Day Challenge

As I said before in this book a body in motion stays in motion, so

momentum is your greatest asset at this point so with that in

mind its important to get you off the best start and start with a

bang. Yes it's 30 day challenge time!

Consistency is key, keep going no matter what.

As Winston Churchill said:

'Never, never, never, never, never give up'

The 30 day challenge is simple but effective so lets start, pulling

no punches Day 1.

Grab your plimsoles and vest we're running.

After your moderate warm up,

Jog/walk(intensity level 4) for 60 seconds

Run/sprint (intensity level 10) 10 seconds

Jog/walk(intensity level 4) for 60 seconds

Run/sprint(intensity level 10) 10 seconds

Jog/walk(intensity level 4) for 60 seconds

Run/sprint (intensity level 10)10 seconds

Jog/walk(intensity level 4) for 60 seconds

Run/sprint 20 seconds

Cool down

Finish

Day 2

Repeat Day 1

Day 3

After your moderate warm up,

Jog/walk(intensity level 4) for 60 seconds

Run/sprint 10 seconds

Jog/walk(intensity level 4) for 60 seconds

Run/sprint 10 seconds

Jog/walk(intensity level 4) for 60 seconds

Run/sprint 10 seconds

Jog/walk(intensity level 4) for 60 seconds

Run/sprint 20 seconds

Jog/walk(intensity level 4) for 60 seconds

Run/sprint 20 seconds

Cool down

Finish

Day 4

Repeat Day 3

Day 5

After your moderate warm up,

Jog/walk(intensity level 4) for 50 seconds

Run/sprint 15 seconds

Jog/walk(intensity level 4) for 50 seconds

Run/sprint 15 seconds

Jog/walk(intensity level 4) for 50 seconds

Run/sprint 15 seconds

Jog/walk(intensity level 4) for 50 seconds

Run/sprint 15 seconds

Jog/walk(intensity level 4) for 50 seconds

Run/sprint 20 seconds

Cool down

Finish

Day 6

Repeat Day 5

Day 7

After your moderate warm up,

Jog/walk(intensity level 4) for 45 seconds

Run/sprint 15 seconds

Jog/walk(intensity level 4) for 45 seconds

Run/sprint 15 seconds

Jog/walk(intensity level 4) for 45 seconds

Run/sprint 15 seconds

Jog/walk(intensity level 4) for 45 seconds

Run/sprint 15 seconds

Jog/walk(intensity level 4) for 45 seconds

Run/sprint 20 seconds

Cool down

Finish

Day 8

Repeat Day 7

Day 9

After your moderate warm up,

Jog/walk(intensity level 4) for 45 seconds

Run/sprint(intensity level 10) 20 seconds

Jog/walk(intensity level 4) for 45 seconds

Run/sprint 20 seconds

Jog/walk(intensity level 4) for 45 seconds

Run/sprint 20 seconds

Jog/walk(intensity level 4) for 45 seconds

Run/sprint 20 seconds

Jog/walk(intensity level 4) for 45 seconds

Run/sprint 25 seconds

Cool down

Finish

Day 10

Rest

Day 11

Repeat Day 9

Day 12

After your moderate warm up,

Jog/walk(intensity level 4) for 40 seconds

Run/sprint(intensity level 10) 20 seconds

Jog/walk(intensity level 4) for 40 seconds

Run/sprint 20 seconds

Jog/walk(intensity level 4) for 40 seconds

Run/sprint 20 seconds

Jog/walk(intensity level 4) for 40 seconds

Run/sprint 20 seconds

Jog/walk(intensity level 4) for 40 seconds

Run/sprint 25 seconds

Cool down

Finish

Day 13

Repeat Day 12

Day 14

After your moderate warm up,

Jog/walk(intensity level 4) for 40 seconds

Run/sprint(intensity level 10) 25 seconds

Jog/walk(intensity level 4) for 40 seconds

Run/sprint 25 seconds

Jog/walk(intensity level 4) for 40 seconds

Run/sprint 25 seconds

Jog/walk(intensity level 4) for 40 seconds

Run/sprint 25 seconds

Jog/walk(intensity level 4) for 40 seconds

Run/sprint 30 seconds

Cool down

Finish

Day 15 HALF WAY! WELL DONE!

Repeat Day 14

Day 16

After your moderate warm up,

Jog/walk(intensity level 4) for 35 seconds

Run/sprint(intensity level 10) 25 seconds

Jog/walk(intensity level 4) for 35 seconds

Run/sprint 25 seconds

Jog/walk(intensity level 4) for 35 seconds

Run/sprint 25 seconds

Jog/walk(intensity level 4) for 35 seconds

Run/sprint 25 seconds

Jog/walk(intensity level 4) for 35 seconds

Run/sprint 30 seconds

Cool down

Finish

Day 17

Repeat Day 16

Day 18

After your moderate warm up,

Jog/walk(intensity level 4) for 35 seconds

Run/sprint(intensity level 10) 30 seconds

Jog/walk(intensity level 4) for 35 seconds

Run/sprint 30 seconds

Jog/walk(intensity level 4) for 35 seconds

Run/sprint 30 seconds

Jog/walk(intensity level 4) for 35 seconds

Run/sprint 30 seconds

Jog/walk(intensity level 4) for 35 seconds

Run/sprint 30 seconds

Cool down

Finish

Day 19

Repeat Day 18

Day 20

After your moderate warm up,

Jog/walk(intensity level 4) for 30 seconds

Run/sprint(intensity level 10) 30 seconds

Jog/walk(intensity level 4) for 30 seconds

Run/sprint 30 seconds

Jog/walk(intensity level 4) for 30 seconds

Run/sprint 30 seconds

Jog/walk(intensity level 4) for 30 seconds

Run/sprint 30 seconds

Jog/walk(intensity level 4) for 30 seconds

Run/sprint 35 seconds

Cool down

Finish

Day 21

Repeat Day 20

Day 22

After your moderate warm up,

Jog/walk(intensity level 4) for 30 seconds

Run/sprint(intensity level 10) 35 seconds

Jog/walk(intensity level 4) for 30 seconds

Run/sprint 35 seconds

Jog/walk(intensity level 4) for 30 seconds

Run/sprint 35 seconds

Jog/walk(intensity level 4) for 30 seconds

Run/sprint 35 seconds

Jog/walk(intensity level 4) for 30 seconds

Run/sprint 35 seconds

Cool down

Finish

Day 23

Repeat Day 22

Day 24

After your moderate warm up,

Jog/walk(intensity level 4) for 25 seconds

Run/sprint(intensity level 10) 35 seconds

Jog/walk(intensity level 4) for 25 seconds

Run/sprint 35 seconds

Jog/walk(intensity level 4) for 25 seconds

Run/sprint 35 seconds

Jog/walk(intensity level 4) for 25 seconds

Run/sprint 35 seconds

Jog/walk(intensity level 4) for 25 seconds

Run/sprint 35 seconds

Cool down

Finish

Day 25

Repeat Day 24

Day 26

After your moderate warm up,

Jog/walk(intensity level 4) for 25 seconds

Run/sprint(intensity level 10) 35 seconds

Jog/walk(intensity level 4) for 25 seconds

Run/sprint 35 seconds

Jog/walk(intensity level 4) for 25 seconds

Run/sprint 35 seconds

Jog/walk(intensity level 4) for 25 seconds

Run/sprint 35 seconds

Jog/walk(intensity level 4) for 25 seconds

Run/sprint 35 seconds

########EXTRA CYCLE#######

Jog/walk(intensity level 4) for 25 seconds

Run/sprint 40 seconds

Cool down

Finish

Day 27

Repeat Day 26

Day 28

After your moderate warm up,

Jog/walk(intensity level 4) for 20 seconds

Run/sprint(intensity level 10) 35 seconds

Jog/walk(intensity level 4) for 20 seconds

Run/sprint 35 seconds

Jog/walk(intensity level 4) for 20 seconds

Run/sprint 35 seconds

Jog/walk(intensity level 4) for 20 seconds

Run/sprint 35 seconds

Jog/walk(intensity level 4) for 20 seconds

Run/sprint 35 seconds

Jog/walk(intensity level 4) for 20 seconds

Run/sprint 40 seconds

Cool down

Finish

Day 29

Repeat Day 28

Day 30

After your moderate warm up,

Jog/walk(intensity level 4) for 20 seconds

Run/sprint(intensity level 10) 35 seconds

Jog/walk(intensity level 4) for 20 seconds

Run/sprint 35 seconds

Jog/walk(intensity level 4) for 20 seconds

Run/sprint 35 seconds

Jog/walk(intensity level 4) for 20 seconds

Run/sprint 35 seconds

Jog/walk(intensity level 4) for 20 seconds

Run/sprint 35 seconds

Jog/walk(intensity level 4) for 20 seconds

Run/sprint 40 seconds

######EXTRA CYCLE######

Jog/walk(intensity level 4) for 20 seconds

Run/sprint 40 seconds

Cool down

Finish

Congratulations, if you've finished and fully completed this 30

challenge you are well on the way to becoming a HIIT pro, now

the future is up to you. Play around with the timings, play

around with your exercises, research some movements that work

for you and the areas you wish to strengthen and develop and

just have fun becoming the person you've always wanted to

become.

Thank you taking the time to download this ebook, if you have enjoyed it please leave a positive review, if you have any areas

you feel I can improve on or wish for more elaboration on please

contact me and let me know. I am always looking for ways to

improve and build on myself and my products.

I really do wish you all the best and sincerely hope you achieve

everything you want in life!

Chapter 16: Treadmill Workout

Running outside is one of the simplest exercises. It is a significant workout, as well, in the high intensity interval workout.

You'll have a healthy heart and body with running. Plus, it's much cheaper than buying a treadmill.

Yet, there will come a time that you will get tired or bored of running. When the winter starts, sprinting will lose its charm on you.

That's the advantage of having a treadmill. It will help you have a consistent exercise even through winter's dark, cold months.

The following are some ideas to change-up your current routine with the use of HIIT:

8-interval sprints

You don't have to make your sprint workouts complicated to be efficient. The most effective workouts are sometimes the simplest ones. Just challenge yourself in each interval and go slow enough to recover between sets so you can push it again each round.

Warm up for 5-10 minutes before you start to use the treadmill. Your muscles need to be adequately warm before sprinting to avoid injury. After warming up, do 8 interval sprinting for half a minute. Recover for 1 minute and 30 seconds. Intensify it by having additional time for sprinting and by decreasing recovery time. You may also sprint faster to increase the challenge. Don't alter all the factors at once. Alter only one factor at a time.

30-second switches

This treadmill workout is all about intensity. You need to have a short and tough interval training workout.

You will sprint for 30 seconds at 12-14mph. You'll get 30 seconds active rest after that before you start sprinting again at the same speed. You need to complete 5 rounds. This workout will only accumulate 5 minutes of your life. Yet, it's really effective.

You can increase the intensity by adding rounds. But if you can't, you don't need to push yourself. Your safety is far more important than having a sexy body.

Strength sprint combo

This is a combination of strength and sprint using a treadmill. You will do a single-leg press for 16 times on each leg onto a treadmill at a 12% incline with 9-10mph. You need to stay at that pace for as long as you can then, jump off to have a rest for 30-60 seconds. Get back on the leg press with the other leg and repeat the instruction.

Hill sprints

Have a solid pace for about 2 minutes with a speed faster than your normal run pace. Your recovery can be 30 seconds to a couple of minutes, depending on fitness level.

If you want something more intense, use a bike or rower for more intense intervals. With the right application, you'll surely enjoy this kind of workout.

Compensated sprints

Sprint workout on a treadmill is an average version of high-intensity interval training. Still, it's one of the best kind of exercise for improving one's strength, speed, endurance and physical performance.

There are compensations which you need to do when sprinting by the use of a treadmill. First, instead of maximal speed, cut it back to 20 or 30% so that you can concentrate on balancing yourself. Second, run as fast as you can when you're slowing down. Lastly, try reducing your recovery or rest time.

It depends on you if you want to buy your own treadmill or go to the gym. Having your own equipment is less important than having time for high intensity interval training. So have a good schedule.

Chapter 17: Workout Routines

Here are some workout routines that you can do. Remember that with these listed exercise, you can virtually mix it up in any order. The main point of doing a HIIT workout is to go very intense so you maximize your workout.

Routine 1:

50 jumping jacks

40 squats

30 switch kicks

20 lunges

10 burpees

20 lunges

30 switch kicks

40 squats

50 jumping jacks

Take a 10 sec rest between each exercise and 1 minute rest between each set. For maximum results, repeat 2-3 times.

Routine 2:

30 squats

40 walking lunges

30 mountain climbers

40 squats

100 jumping jacks

40 walking lunges

50 second wall squat

40 calf raises

Take a 10 sec rest between each exercise and 1 minute rest between each set. For maximum results, repeat 2-3 times.

Routine 3:

15 squats

30 bicycle crunches

10 pushups

30 sec plank

20 sit-ups

20 side crunches

Take a 10 sec rest between each exercise and 1 minute rest between each set. For maximum results, repeat 2-3 times.

Routine 4:

Squat jumps

Push ups

Split lunge jumps

Tricep dips

Mountain climbers

Bicycle crunches

Complete each exercise for 45 seconds, then rest for 15 seconds. Rest for 1 minute after each set and repeat 2-3 times for maximum results.

Routine 5:

Jumping lunges

High knees

Mountain climbers

Suicide drills

Heisman

Burpees

Jumping jacks

Squats

Complete each exercise for 30 seconds, rest for 10 seconds. Rest for 1 minute after each set and repeat 2-3 times for maximum results.

Routine 6:

Squat jumps

Pushups

Skaters

Jump rope

Jumping jacks

Plank hold

Jumping lunges

Complete each exercise for 30 seconds, rest for 10 seconds. Rest for 1 minute after each set and repeat 2-3 times for maximum results.

As you can tell, you can see some repetition in the exercises, but this is because they have been proven to work and it makes you sweat up! Play around with the exercise and create your own workout. Understand that it doesn't matter what you do, but as long as you stay active, you will shed the weight in no time

Conclusion

I hope this book was able to help you learn more about HIIT.

The next step is to put this information to use, and begin high intensity interval training! Remember to assess your goals and current level of fitness before beginning. Design a training routine that fits your requirements, and get to work!

Also, if you haven't exercised in a while, are over 40, have any pre-existing health issues, or are on any medication, remember to first consult a medical professional before you begin HIIT. As the name suggests, it is intense and you definitely do not want to over do it!

Thank you and good luck!

www.ingramcontent.com/pod-product-compliance
Lightning Source LLC
Chambersburg PA
CBHW062134020426
42335CB00013B/1214